© **Copyright 2021 - All rights reserved.**

The content contained within this book may not be reproduced, duplicated, or transmitted without direct written permission from the author or the publisher.

Under no circumstances will any blame or legal responsibility be held against the publisher, or author, for any damages, reparation, or monetary loss due to the information contained within this book, either directly or indirectly.

Legal Notice:

This book is copyright protected. It is only for personal use. You cannot amend, distribute, sell, use, quote, or paraphrase any part of the content within this book without the author or publisher's consent.

Disclaimer Notice:

Please note the information contained within this document is for educational and entertainment purposes only. All effort has been executed to present accurate, up-to-date, reliable, complete information. No warranties of any kind are declared or implied. Readers acknowledge that the author is not engaged in the rendering of legal, financial, medical, or professional advice. The content within this book has been derived from various sources. Please consult a licensed professional before attempting any techniques outlined in this book.

By reading this document, the reader agrees that under no circumstances is the author responsible for any losses, direct or indirect, that are incurred due to the use of the information in this document, including, but not limited to, errors, omissions, or inaccuracies.

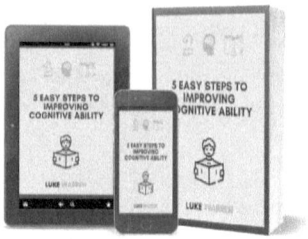

As a special gift to you, included with your purchase of this book are my 5 Easy Steps to Improving Cognitive Ability. These Steps will help instill methodical thinking into your subconscious and provide you with the advantage of gaining transferrable skills through learning psychological, academic tricks.

Please visit methodicalmindset.com to download or https://www.facebook.com/groups/MethodicalMindset and click join.

Thank you.

TESTOSTERONE AND DEPRESSION

A PERSPECTIVE ON MALE MENTAL HEALTH:
UNDISCLOSED BY MAINSTREAM MEDIA

LUKE WARREN

ABOUT THE AUTHOR

Luke Warren has a formal educational background in computer science, but his real passion lies in the art of systematic and rational thinking. He is an autodidact and a polymath whose thirst for knowledge has led him down an extended learning and self-studying road. Early in his life, Luke and his family discovered his ability to condense immensely complex tasks into a structured art form. Because of his innate gift, he has always been passionate about helping others unlock their critical thinking and rationality potential. He learned at a young age that with just a few essential rules and well-placed prompts, he could assist anyone who wanted to enhance their cognitive and cerebral skills regardless of the situation.

Luke's tenacity in his passion for helping others through learning and education can be attributed to his upbringing in Northern England. He was raised as an only child in a single-parent household and found himself devoted to knowledge rather than sports, or other entities children of similar age were interested in. He understood that he couldn't use brute strength or athleticism to outmanoeuvre life's obstacles. Instead, he had to rely on his intellect and mental wit to uplift himself and become successful. He acquired a BSc in computing and engineering and has had many years of experience as a full-stack web developer. The nature of his profession helped sharpen his capacity for thinking by adopting principles from artificial intelligence. Luke discovered that he could borrow logical properties from artificial intelligence and apply it to everyday thinking. This discovery led him to become highly efficient and conscientious with his work while also maximising his cognitive potential.

Luke has taken it upon himself to help anyone who needs guidance in logical and systematic thinking. He understands the importance of these skills because they have helped him make some of the most significant decisions in his life. Whether in business negotiations, interviews, meetings, investment pitches, or University debates, he has always relied on these skills to help him flourish and find success. Now, he wants you, the reader, to find the same success with these skills also.

AUTHOR'S NOTE

Hi there,

Firstly, thank you for purchasing. This publication has been many months in the making, and I am so pleased to finally release the product providing you with the value and knowledge you deserve. I am desperate to help men like yourself, and if you can get any value from this short read, that will make my day much better. This book highlights a general exploration into hormone-connected depression; if you are depressed, or feeling low, then hopefully, I can provide some way to a feasible explanation. I firmly believe in problem and solution, cause and effect. For every action, there is a reaction, said Newton. Therefore, I want to apply these practices to the situations we confront daily as men. It is no secret that male mental health has recently become primarily neglected in favour of more "popular" or brand-friendly causes. However, our response to this neglect is what makes us iron-willed and forged from metaphorical steel. We have carried countries on our backs through wars and famines, from biblical times to today. Picking up this book proves you do not think like the rest; you think outside the box and are happy not conforming with mainstream rhetoric. I am here for you and only you. I want to provide you with an alternative to mental health repair by explaining the hypothesis, which I think is one of the leading causes of male depression. I want to help you get better.

Hopefully, you gain everlasting knowledge and a reprieve from what legacy media usually perpetuates; I hope you can gain value from my work. If you have a spare 60 seconds, then a book review on Amazon would be hugely appreciated as it only helps more young and older men in the future.

Thank you,

Luke

WHY AM I WRITING THIS BOOK?

Hi There, thank you for your purchase. It means an awful lot to me, as you are obviously interested in the hypothesis I'm about to present. Therefore, we have some things in common. In this short book, what is discussed is not addressed within the mainstream media, especially not here in the UK. Why this is the case, I'm not quite sure? Perhaps lack of financial recourse, lack of interest within this scope, or maybe it's an easily fixed problem and does not meet the interests of the powers that be? Nevertheless, I believe hormone treatment may save many issues for our National Health Service here in the UK, and potentially, it may make financial sense. It's possible that prescribing exogenous hormones may save more money in other medical fields by releasing financial burdens on departments such as mental health and perhaps cardiology, as there are a host of health issues that come with inherent low testosterone.

I hope to offer you, the reader, some help and guidance if you're currently in a challenging position in life. Hopefully, you've picked up this book at just the right time, and it can be the antidote to what you're searching for. I do not want to promise too much, but I guarantee this book has been written with its primary focus at all times being on the mental and psychological wellbeing of men like yourself in mind. That is my promise to you, and this promise is to all men, so if you're younger and reading this, then the hypothesis presented is not exclusive to the older male as it may be perceived depression leading to suicide is most common in men aged 40+.

So, before we begin, I must state, I'm not a doctor or a medical expert. I'm pretty much a regular guy, like yourself, who isn't happy with the attention put on men's mental health. Not that men's mental health doesn't get attention, there are some fantastic charities such as CALM, Male Voiced & much more. But it's what the attention focus' on, I believe lacks scope. Most mental health charities, therapists, and psychologists constantly focus on cause & effect. Trauma, for example, is subject to much focus as a reason for feeling depressed, and that's fine, but many times the obsessiveness over one singular aspect of cause and effect just doesn't cut it for me. I'm confident British society either ignores or plainly, just does not know enough about hormones and the role hormones play in one's physical and mental performance. This may be the case for women, too & their oestrogen levels, but for this book, I'll be focusing on men & testosterone.

Finally, I will be citing British sources for this book and using predominantly British examples for my publication. The reasons for this are because I'm British myself, and I feel the attention hormones receive in the USA are already ahead of British Medical Associations by some years. However, this book will still be highly pertinent to many men across the pond also. So please, be aware, everything is entirely relevant no matter where you're located.

1

MY INTEREST IN THE ENDOCRINE SYSTEM

I must've been aged 19 or 20 when I first discovered my grandfather attempted to take his own life in the mid-1980s. My mum says she woke one morning to find him unconscious on the kitchen floor, and it was later discovered this was due to an attempted overdose. I can only imagine how horrible the experience must've been for all involved. It was a tough time in Northern England during that decade; unemployment reached its highest point since Trading Economics started capturing employment statistics in 1971. Margaret Thatcher became prime minister in 1979 and was a very fiscally prudent leader. It appears economic outsourcing and privatisation of some fields such as transport & manual labour exports may have directly exacerbated a sharp turn in unemployment around that period, specifically impacting the working class. I wasn't born at the time, and I'm not here to provide a political opinion, but with Grandad out of work and aged 50+, it must have felt like there was not much to live for at the time.

Keep in mind; this is mid-1980s Great Britain; there is

no internet and no social media, meaning jobs that become available are either printed in the local newspaper or posted on a job's board at the local Job Centre. It must've felt like people were competing for scraps. You can imagine with more time on people's hands, with mouths to feed and families to provide for; depression would've gripped many men at that time due to financial responsibility historically leaning on the man of the household. Like my grandfather, I expect many from that era to have lived during the Second World War and to have developed a particular "battle-hardened" mentality with life being more brutal throughout the war and the years that followed in many places across the west. However, it's also acknowledged that mental health awareness has been a slow burner; talking about depression and mental health has largely only come to light from the mid to late 90s, particularly within men, I find.

This may mean for my grandfather and other men of that era that depression and male depression, more so, is not something the public was made aware of initially and throughout the 1980s, specifically. The acknowledgment depression and men's mental health have had in the last few years is fantastic.

Still, I am confident an overall lack of observation within the male realm of depression may be occurring, and this is what I will be delving into. I'm happy to say my grandfather survived his attempted suicide and that episode; he was treated in hospital and made a full recovery. He ended up living the rest of his life until age 90, in March 2018 until he, unfortunately, succumbed to cancer.

So why am I telling you this? Well, for one, suicide is not something I have thought about in either committing the act or thought about it through curiosity either. I've always been a person who has remained content throughout life, and not many things have bothered me. However, a couple of years back, I read an article and viewed an ONS (Office of National Statistics) stat that most suicides occur in men, and the highest singular stat of suicide victims occurs in men aged 40+. This correlated with my grandfather and made me think that it's easy to suggest baron periods in an economy are easy to connect to depression and, therefore, suicide. Although socio-economic downturns contribute towards depression, and by extension, suicide, this has compelled me to discover if there are additional correlations that contribute to male suicides. What if these variables cannot be seen, and possibly they are not mental causes for depression but physical causes of depression? If so, can these physical causes be potentially prevented and cured?

Of course, having job security, money in our pockets, and the social aspect of interacting with colleagues every day helps to alleviate depression and loneliness. But does this mean depression is always there? Is depression something that lurks beneath our exteriors, and only a few factors have to align simultaneously, allowing pressure to build perfectly, and we finally crack? Was my grandfather similar to myself, perhaps? Got along with his life completely fine, and eventually, the pressure was too much? This may be the case, but we also know depression hits the richest and the most famous. Linkin Park lead singer Chester Bennington, Celebrity chef Anthony Bourdaine & Fashion Designer Alexander McQueen prove depression is a phenomenon that is not exclusive to working-class men in society, and it does not discriminate.

Understandably, throughout all of this, depression and suicides are not exclusive to men either. Sadly, this is the case for women also. But why does it seem its exclusivity impacts men of a particular age bracket? And far more than women? According to Samaritans' website, in the UK, Men aged 45 - 49 still have the highest rate of suicides. Male suicide rates even increased for this group during 2018, and it's interesting to think what the figures may present come to the end of the pandemic. For you, the reader, I aim to deliver a hypothesis I believe is possibly being missed for many cases of male depression. In the UK, you may book an appointment with your doctor concerning negative thoughts you're experiencing, or suddenly your mood has become particularly deflated. You find yourself in a rut for a few weeks, you cannot get out of bed, have no energy, and you become apathetic to most situations. You visit your doctor, who will likely be part of the NHS (National Health Service), describe your feelings, and the solution provided by a doctor is usually; CBT therapy, talking to a private therapist, or being prescribed antidepressants such as sertraline (Zoloft) or fluoxetine (Prozac).

This is fine if there is a genuine chemical imbalance in the brain, but overall, this is lazy. It's a centralised way of treating the problem through a one size fits all method. I am not criticising the NHS because what they do is terrific, but the powers that be appear to act idly when treating cases such as mental health in men, and the evidence more needs to be done is displayed in the statistics of male suicide rates. The national health service focuses on reactive health care within the general public rather than preventative care. This is not the fault of individual doctors or nurses, but something the UK government & health secretary should investigate instead. It should not be the responsibility of the NHS to be pioneers of diagnosis to such problems. Still, when we see the average UK workplace, GP practises, and general hospitals, there are many posters, intranet bulletins, and staff awareness days concerning our mental health. Yet, its acknowledgement and treatment remain too holistic.

Now I reiterate the NHS themselves and mental health charities such as CALM & Male Voiced are fantastic. Still, the general focus remains on mental wellbeing, talking about our feelings, and ultimately this will go some way to solving our problems, etc. Of course, this will work for many men as there may be a traumatic experience that causes their depression, but what about men who are depressed and there is no apparent connection for this depression? The NHS and mental health charities are not looking at the aspects in a surgical approach to find the cause and solution of male mental health issues. For me, the process is very generalised within the media. When considering potential causes of depressive mood in men, the dialogue needs to shift its direction and become more methodical. Otherwise, you have to go looking outside the proverbial box if you want solutions that aren't visible in the UK mainstream.

2

HYPOTHESIS

So what solutions am I talking about? Well, I used to be passionate about the gym, as cliché as it sounds, and I'm sure you were at some point too. However, I became highly dedicated to attending the gym, almost addicted from approximately ages 21 to 27. I'd attend up to 4 or 5 times per week with my friend David, almost ritualistically, and I was extremely strict with my diet. However, I encountered a problem that occurs to many of us. I plateaued and could not burn additional fat or gain muscle, etc., depending on my regime. After many months I became emotionally deflated as a consequence. My best years of peak performance were passing by, and I did not see the results I had worked so hard for. This led me to investigate why I was not getting results; other people looked great, but not me. I started researching online, reading forums, looking at different studies, and not before long. I'd ventured down the internet rabbit hole of personal anecdotes & people's experiences of using PEDS (Performing Enhancing Drugs). I became interested in this myself and started to explore different anabolic properties;

Testosterone, Deca-Durabolin, Nandrolone, Primobolan, Trenbolone, to name a few. I became frustrated with my lack of progress, and steroids were sounding like a feasible option. My interest in this area was to solely maintain a solid physique, nothing ridiculous such as Captain America's transformation, just something presentable to show off at the beach. Looking back, it's clear to see my problems at the time were born out of vanity mostly. I'd spent many years being the fat kid, and I was desperate to be the opposite of that. I craved it.

Forward to now, and I can say I never actually consumed PEDS. I'd researched & discovered information about them and remain very much open-minded to the idea. I don't knock anyone using them as it is their business. But I did come very close to venturing down that road, leading me to have my blood tested privately. The blood tests I ordered checked my free and total testosterone as suggested by nearly every forum I had come across; *"you need to get your bloods tested," "you're training blind if you haven't tested your T levels."* In this search for self-medication, the common denominator was always the repeated rhetoric of *"you need to be running a baseline testosterone dose if you're gonna jump on peds."* Being very disappointed in my gym progress led me to discover the importance of testosterone and other metabolic properties that occur endogenously within the body.

Apart from being disappointed in my physique, perhaps it stems from body dysmorphia, I don't' know, but I was actually very content and happy with life as a whole. No mental health issues, slight anxiety, nothing out of the ordinary, but reading forums, watching videos, etc., the narrative all repeated one thing; *"Get your T levels tested."*

So, I followed people's advice on forums and began looking at how I could book in for a blood test that would precisely measure free and total testosterone. I assumed this would be the norm and expected this to be a regular occurrence that doctors encounter from most men and something they check for regularly. But no. Upon attempting to have my hormones tested, a doctor I spoke with advised this was not something made available unless I am experiencing severe depression or a genuine cause for concern is present, such as an immediate impact on general health. As I say, I wasn't depressed, I've always been relatively content, and I was very physically healthy. Based on this, I had no chance of obtaining a hormone check through the NHS, and this is what happened. I find this extremely disappointing, considering the rhetoric perpetuated by such governing bodies and healthcare institutions. To be honest, whether it be advice on how to deal with mental health issues or preventative care physically, UK Government and UK public health continually advise people to talk with someone concerning depression. I understand the NHS are emergency care specialists. Still, when I tried to take care of myself and seek medical evidence pertaining to my endocrine system in preventative measures, psychological and physical health suddenly did not matter.

This is 2017, so the NHS may have changed its approach in acknowledging hormone depletion within men, but a quick look at its website implies it is not the case. The suggestion of the cause for testosterone depletion is lifestyle & external factors, which are accurate, however. But you end up with a chicken & egg scenario and a negative feedback loop. Does natural low testosterone cause low mood and depression? Or do external factors cause testosterone to crash? Can low testosterone be inherent to any male, at any age, of any weight? And even if they feel physically great, can depletion of this hormone be natural or inherently low to begin with?

That's ultimately the aim of this book; highlighting the probable cause of male depression and other feelings that can afflict many men of all ages: a low sex drive, lack of determination, and apathy towards finding purpose. I genuinely believe having an innate low testosterone level can contribute to these factors rather than external factors causing testosterone to become low, especially combined with the natural decline in testosterone occurring in men around age 30.

3

MEASURING TESTOSTERONE

Now, this hypothesis follows the evidence. It follows the exploration of my research in discovering my personal testosterone levels. In 2016, after being rejected to have my hormones tested by the NHS, I sought private examination; I had my blood tested with a company called Medichecks, based in the UK. At this time, I was aged 25, 5 ft 9, and weighed 170lb. That's a pretty healthy height-to-weight ratio, especially considering I had been powerlifting for 18 months to two years and ate a primarily healthy lifestyle consisting of lean proteins & carbohydrates. I also played football two times per week, and cardio/stamina was pretty good too. I was physically fit; you would not think there was anything wrong with me when looking at me.

So, I researched the average testosterone levels for men and the average for a male my age. The USA and UK measure their levels differently. The USA measures ng/dL (nanogram per decilitre) compared to the UK, which measures nmol/L (nanomole per litre). The USA uses higher overall numbers, in the hundreds, which directly converts to a smaller number in the UK. For example, a testosterone presence of 600 ng/dL in blood using the United States' metrics converts to 20.8 nmol/dL in the UK. According to Balance My Hormones and other scientific literature, it is suggested an absolute natural peak in testosterone should be at approximately aged 20 in males. The caveat when researching healthy levels occurs due to most data persisting in maintaining a healthy "range" between testosterone measurements rather than giving a specific example, i.e., *"18 nmol/L of total testosterone is healthy and what you should aim for"*. The range most medical data uses is far too broad as you can have healthy testosterone levels on paper yet still experience negative consequences of low testosterone. The literature was more accurate, providing a specific reading and stating; 18 nmol/L (mentioned above) as a target number for healthy hormone levels. That would be far more beneficial and enable men to assess how hormonally healthy they are, rather than having a man score in the healthy range from 8.64 nmol to 29 nmol, as this reading remains pretty vague. If you're below 15 nmol/L, it's still very feasible you will experience side effects of low testosterone.

As men age, testosterone will naturally decline year after year, approximately at a rate of 1%. You can probably guess some of the symptoms that correlate to low testosterone levels as we get older. Harvard Medical School researchers suggest some of the things that decline within men due to testosterone decreasing are; memory, muscle mass, bone density, and our red blood cell count becomes lower also. Sexual ardour declines, and body fat increases.

Harvard researchers continue and advise testosterone prescription therapy may mitigate and even reverse each of these changes.

As mentioned previously, the advised levels of a healthy testosterone range for men in the UK, as of December 2018, are 8.64 nmol/L – 29 nmol/L. To me, that's quite a broad range. Of course, the cut-off point must occur at a particular digit. However, a 30-year-old male with a total testosterone level of 9 nmol/L will still potentially suffer from the properties induced by hypogonadism, potentially leading to depression. The problem occurs due to the National Health Service and mainstream media not acknowledging that low testosterone can directly impact one's feelings of deflation, nihilism, or apathy.

Firstly, the individual will not have their hormones tested due to male endocrine health problems not being a significant concern for public health entities. Secondly, male endocrine health is not perpetuated by the mainstream media. Therefore, as men, we may likely remain unaware of the impact hypogonadal properties can have on mental health. If this is the first time you have heard of this connection, then not to worry. It's almost by design the general public is told how to deal with mental health issues, such as talking to someone, opening up to friends, consuming anti-depressants, etc. I reiterate; mental health treatment has come on leaps and bounds but remains very singular symptom-minded as it only focuses on repairing the mind as the solution. You can treat hormones, gut microbiome, and many other physical properties within the body, which can alleviate depression. I believe the mainstream is playing catch up when we talk about endocrinology, particularly in men. A lot of information already exists helping women when we consider menopause, menstrual cycles, but not much literature on the subject is available to men.

Now, from personal experience, as a male, if you want a blood test that measures your hormones and endocrine system, then be prepared to fight tooth and nail as it's doubtful to happen. However, on the miracle, the NHS agrees to test your hormones; if you're in the range of 9 nmol/L (mentioned previously), you will be classed in the "healthy" testosterone range. This means public health will see no issues with your hormonal balance, even though your testosterone is deficient at 9 nmol/L; but, by public health definition, no problems exist within hormone deficiencies at this level. Following a "healthy" result, the total focus then shifts to prescribing anti-depressants, attending therapy, etc., if you are experiencing severe depression.

This is a grave error, in my opinion. Though this measurement of 9 nmol/ L will pass as healthy, these are the testosterone levels of a man in his mid-40s to 50s, yet these levels regularly appear in younger males. However, because Public Health maintains a decline in testosterone is natural in men around the age of 30+. Public Health sees no problem and does not attempt to remedy the individual from a hormone-focused perspective; instead, they try to heal the mind to alleviate depression.

Considering this, is it a coincidence that most cases of suicide occur in men at the age of 40 +? Perhaps there may be a direct correlation between low testosterone &

suicide at this age? It's important to understand that testosterone does decline in men, as mentioned previously. However, some men under 30 already have almost hypogonadism levels of the hormone, and public health still maintains this is healthy if they are within range; 8.64 - 29 nmol/L.

There are two issues here; issue 1: We have a collection of young men in the west with innate low testosterone levels, issue 2: We have the natural decline of testosterone occurring within men from ages 30+. Both groupsets can suffer from mental health problems and severe depression. Yet, minimal investigation transpires by public health associating inherent low testosterone in younger men to depression—the same when relating testosterone declining in older men as a link to depression and suicide also. If we have a male suffering from depression and anxiety, and blood is taken measuring the subject's hormones, showing results of low testosterone levels and he is labelled "healthy" on paper, our subject will proceed to appear healthy from a hormonal perspective, and no further investigations into his endocrine system will occur. This laissez-faire attitude is unlikely to heal our subject's mental health problems and therefore, the medicine provided is likely to be therapy, and a prescription of anti-depressants, all the while, the subject's hormone levels remain shot.

You may ask, if anti-depressants and therapy sessions will not alleviate depression, then what will? I believe this comes in the form of therapeutic testosterone provided to the body exogenously; testosterone replacement therapy (TRT), but this is only when adequate avenues have been explored. Ultimately though, I believe this discussion needs to be brought to public attention and should not be so taboo, as its only aim is to assist men who are in this position and have not felt like themselves in a long time.

Suppose we have two male subjects, both aged 25, for example. Subject A has testosterone levels of 20 nmol/L. Subject B has testosterone levels of 10 nmol/L. There is a massive disparity within these levels for context, but public health will declare both males in the healthy range, and yet subject B is far likelier to experience mental health problems. Subject A feels fantastic and amazing most days, doesn't get depressed, and is reasonably mature about most situations, and responds very well to physical exercise and diet – a higher total testosterone level means nutrients become more bioavailable in the body.

Subject B, however, constantly feels melancholic and has a persistent nihilistic perspective on the world. He continually feels irritated and is relatively short-fused also. Subject B speaks to his GP and is prescribed anti-depressants. As mentioned, it's unlikely there will even be an investigation into his hormonal levels as both patient and doctor will likely follow the mainstream narrative when treating mental health and depression. I must add, it's not guaranteed that therapeutic doses of exogenous testosterone will cure subject B's low mood and despondent behaviour, but is it not at the very least worth exploring as a means of treatment? Rather than continual diagnoses of depression amongst young men?

. . .

Of course, with an increase in testosterone comes an increase in overall muscle mass; there is a considerable boost physically for men, not just mentally. However, many men who are in a similar position to subject B will remain unaware of low testosterone as a potential cause of their depression. It's unlikely to have been previously highlighted as an issue. Therefore, the persistent tonic of anti-depressive drugs will likely prolong this cycle of extremely low-level hormones, and in some individuals, perpetual sequences of up and down mood swings, the case for many men in western society these days.

4

PROBLEMS WITH DIAGNOSIS & ANTIDOTE

When we consider the broad range of "healthy" in male hormones, this presents two problems. Problem one; It's unlikely that our hypothetical patient, subject B, with a testosterone level of 10 nmol/L suffering from depression, will be tested for hypogonadism or even have his hormones measured. This does not appear to be in the interests of the UK Public Health & Government to explore. If we go down this avenue, our patient will likely be issued with prescription anti-depressants, be told to "eat well," and may well be assigned cognitive behavioural therapy (CBT), as mentioned previously. The diagnosis of his problems will likely be treated with mental health at the fore. There will be a low probability our patient's endocrine system will be explored for the potential cause of any issues. This means It is unlikely his total testosterone will improve in the following months, and our subject's mental health may improve through using anti-depressants, but it may not. In this case, our subject will continually remain unaware of issues that may be being caused by a low total testosterone range.

Problem number two is the rare situation where our male case study living with 10 nmol/L of total testosterone does have his hormones checked by public health services. In this case, our subject will pass with flying colours, and it will look like his hormones are in balance because he sits in that "healthy" range between 8.64 - 29 nmol/L, albeit our subject is at the bottom of the healthy scale with a paltry score of 10/29. At this point, no further treatment on his hormones will take place, and medical staff will likely progress to using different antidotes to alleviate our subject's mental struggles, as mentioned previously.

This means when evaluating a healthy hormonal range in men, I believe the traditional measures in practice are too low, to begin with. This will likely induce a false sense of security within the test subject. He will believe he is hormonally healthy and may continue to seek other solutions to combat mental health. An average male aged approximately 30 years of age, such as our example, will be passed as healthy with a presence of 10 nmol/L of testosterone in the blood. For me, this is a significant cause for concern. The scale needs to be moved a few places to the right. A better range and using the same scale would be to start at, at least 15 nmol/L – 30/35 nmol/L. I think it's in the best interests of the powers, that be, to keep this scale at its current measurements, and the same for the American scale when using ng/dL. I don't exactly know why this is the case. Still, as I said near the beginning of the book, there seems to be a collective apathy towards hormonal deficiencies within men or a collective lack of knowledge on the subject.

5

MY ANECDOTAL EXPERIENCE

So as a 25-year-old male, I had my testosterone tested privately. After researching, I expected to possess levels around the range of 20 nmol/L. Considering I was 25, exercised and weight trained regularly, never smoked, and only drunk alcohol a couple of times a month, nothing excessive. When I finally received my results, three days after my initial blood test, I was shocked to find I was displaying testosterone levels measured at 6.7 nmol/L. That's an American equivalent of 193.24 ng/dL—basically, the levels of a 70-year-old man or someone suffering from hypogonadism. However, I had no symptoms of this, physically or mentally.

This shocked me to the core at the time as it just didn't make logical sense. How can I bench up to 250lb naturally, weighing 170lb, and have the hormone levels of a pensioner? The test date was May 2016, and I maintained I wasn't going to do anything drastic based on my results, PED-wise, I thought looking into external injections of testosterone may be a knee-jerk reaction. I waited a further year, and at the start of 2017, I started eating a vegetarian diet. One year later, this time May 2017, I re-tested myself, this time aged 26, my total testosterone measured 10.94 nmol/L

So, my total testosterone had increased by a measurement of 4 nmol/dL in 12 months, but the overall level was still deficient and barely healthy. Now If this had been my first hormone test, I might have assumed this was down to eating something the day before, not enough sleep, maybe even it's a one-off, and I can work with these levels to get myself up to a 22/23 nmol level, something respectable for my age group. Any theories of this were put to bed when I had my third test; however, this time, I measured my free testosterone and my blood proteins, such as SHBG (sexual hormone-binding globulin).

SHBG is a protein that transports sex hormones such as testosterone & oestrogen in the blood. It's measured using the same metrics; nmol/L. A healthy range is 18.3 – 54.1 nmol/L. My SBHG measured at 19 nmol. Again, I'm at the bottom end of the scale, which correlated to my latest test in December 2018, presenting a total testosterone level of 10.4 nmol/L. However, with low SHBG, my available testosterone should be bio-available in the body to use in theory. A higher measurement of SHBG would mean hormones are far more likely to bind with androgens and would not be available for the body to use. However, with my natural levels so low in total and free testosterone, there is little to work with, and my hormonal pattern seems consistently low. When comparing my results from 2017 to

2018, that represents a decrease of 0.5 nmol of total testosterone after an initial rise of 4 nmol the previous year. Also, my free testosterone measured 0.26. The range for free testosterone is a lot lower than total. Free testosterone is calculated at 0.2 – 0.62 nmol/dL, So again, I'm significantly on the low end of the scale. By now, it's pretty evident that my testosterone is naturally at a low level. One comment from the private doctor, Dr. Kamali, after my third test read:

"Thank you, Luke, for the information you've provided. I can see your testosterone has been low in the past. If you are experiencing symptoms, I recommend discussing this further with your GP. Your oestradiol levels are within the normal range. You have normal levels of proteins. Best Wishes, Dr. Hamed Kamali"

My latest blood results measuring my hormone range, aged 29. Dated 24/03/2021:

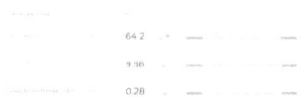

The issue presented here leaves me in a predicament; what am I supposed to do from here? Do I just endure these low levels for the next 10 – 15 years? Perhaps I will remain fine and mentally sound. But what if depression hits me at an older age? Am I simply waiting for the inevitable to occur?

Maybe if I remained unaware of such low levels and in the future went to a GP and discussed low mood, depressive thoughts I may be having, will any GP even test my hormones? Right at this moment, the answer is no, as I am classed as hormonally healthy. It would be far more likely that I am prescribed anti-depressants in the UK as I am not eligible for testosterone replacement therapy, even though we can see how hormonally deficient I am. My worry is how many other men are similar to myself yet remain unaware. I believe this is where the error occurs, which makes me think there may be a consistent misdiagnosis of depression within men.

This issue is close to my heart because there is a history of depression in both my families, especially within the men, and I know they have not had their hormones tested as I have. To be honest, hormone crashes or inherently low testosterone levels do not occur to be a factor for most of the male population within the UK. This is not their fault. As previously mentioned, it's something that public health and mainstream media do not perpetuate to the general public, it's not advertised in the mainstream, but depression and mental health disorders are continually displayed within British health services and most British workplaces. I hope to change that, and again I reiterate, not to discourage people from seeking help for mental health problems, I hope to change the one size fits all diagnosis within men. Therefore, I hope this book brings you some awareness of the effects hormone deficiencies may have on male mental health.

6

A CASE FOR TESTOSTERONE OVER ANTI-DEPRESSANTS

A healthy testosterone level in men is associated with a happy and overall positive mood, generally according to Dr. Andreas Walther, Ph.D., a co-author of research undertaken at Dresden University. Walther continues; a feeling of wellbeing and cognitive clarity occurs when men are supplemented with a therapeutic dose of testosterone.

In the journal; Jama Psychiatry, Walther et al. report their review of 27 random-controlled trials undertaken since 2000 involving 1,890 men. Some of the studies investigated men with a testosterone deficiency, and others examined men without hormonal deficiencies. Not all studies involved men diagnosed with depressive disorder, but some did include men with symptoms of depression. Other participants underwent treatments with established anti-depressants or therapy.

Intriguingly, Walther & the other researchers discovered an improvement in depression and depressive symptoms in men supplied with exogenous testosterone compared to the men who did not receive hormone treatment. Results from seven of the studies with necessary data revealed when comparing therapeutic testosterone treatment with a placebo, the probabilities of participants having a 50% or greater decrease in their depressive symptoms improved by 130% when testosterone was supplied. This resulted in the team advising that testosterone supplementation could claim parity with the efficacy of established anti-depressants.

The team also found that when a testosterone dosage was at least 500mg per week and the disparity in symptoms between participants was low, and the treatment was linked to significant reductions in depressive symptoms. Also, the researchers advise benefits can be seen within six weeks of beginning treatment, and both younger and older men could experience mood improvements. They say the review did not show that the benefits were confined to men who had a testosterone deficiency, to begin with, or who had a particular severity of depression.

From what I've studied myself, 500mg of testosterone per week is exceptionally high for a therapeutic dose. I've seen anecdotal evidence of someone vlogging their experience with testosterone replacement therapy (TRT). They seem very content at a low dose of 140mg per week. I expect this will vary amongst individuals, but 500mg of testosterone per week appears to be advised for some steroid cycles. That's an entirely different topic, however. Still, regardless of whether you are suffering from low testosterone levels biologically, 200mg per week should do the trick in alleviating depression and helping you feel good again.

. . .

It's also worth noting; testosterone comes in different forms, known as esters. Esters are simply the oil the testosterone is contained within. Therefore, you may hear of testosterone cypionate, testosterone enanthate, or testosterone propionate. This just means how frequently you have to inject, basically. Each ester/oil will play its role in deploying the exogenous testosterone into your blood, which will impact the frequency of pinning. Enanthate, for example, may only require an injection once every five days. This is due to enanthate and its properties slowly metabolising and releasing the exogenous testosterone within your system. However, Sustanon 250 is often the version used when prescribing a TRT dose.

7
METHODS THAT BOOST TESTOSTERONE NATURALLY

Boron Supplementation

Up to 6mg, a day of boron mineral consumption can improve the conversion of total testosterone to free testosterone through its metabolic pathway by up to 30%. After one week of boron supplementation of 6 mg/d, a study by Naghii et al. of healthy males (n = 8) found a significant increase in free testosterone, rising from an average of 11.83 pg/mL to 15.18 pg/mL; with substantial decreases in oestradiol, dropping from 42.33 pg/mL to 25.81 pg/mL almost a 50% decrease. Approximately 98% of testosterone molecules are bound to proteins in the blood, principally to SHBG, and are not bioavailable because bound hormones cannot exit capillaries. Therefore, the elevation of unbound free testosterone seen with boron supplementation may have significant advantages, particularly in aging men where levels of SHBG increase and levels of free testosterone decrease.

Sleep

Testosterone levels increase as you sleep and decrease the longer you stay awake. When sleeping, the highest testosterone levels occur during REM sleep, the period late in the cycle helping to replenish the body and mind. That is why it does not take long for lousy quality sleep to disrupt your testosterone production. One study showed after eight days of 5.5 hours of sleep or less per night, participants displayed an average of 10-15% decrease in testosterone production.

Exercise and strength training

Both stimulate growth hormone and testosterone release, irrespective of age. A study showing obese men regularly exercised, increased testosterone levels more compared to losing weight with calorie restriction.

Ashwagandha

A herb regularly used in Ayurvedic medicine promotes youthful vigour, enhances muscle strength and endurance, and promotes overall health. One study investigated the effects ashwagandha had in overweight men with mild fatigue. After eight weeks of taking ashwagandha, there was a 14.7% increase in testosterone. Another study showed that taking ashwagandha was associated with increased testosterone levels, and they speculate it is due to its stress-relieving effects.

Stress Management

Vital to maintaining adequate testosterone levels. When you experience stressful events, it can cause changes in your testosterone levels. When experiencing psychological stress, it can cause your serum testosterone levels to decrease. This is because cortisol, the primary stress hormone released from the adrenal cortex in a stressful situation, suppresses testosterone formation. Stress management starts with detecting the stress source. Determining the source of stress begins with looking closely at your habits, attitude, and excuses.

Increase Vitamin D Absorption

Low circulating vitamin D levels are related to lower total testosterone levels. Researchers found that this vitamin can also help maintain optimal testosterone levels. One study showed blood samples that were taken from 800 middle-aged men. The results showed that 68% of them had low vitamin D levels. However, only 11% of the deficient participants in vitamin D were supplemented with vitamin D to correct the deficiency. The men who did not consume a vitamin D supplement continue to have low testosterone levels, while those who supplemented had higher testosterone levels. Follow up with your doctor to ask about having your levels checked.

MY ADVICE FOR YOU

So, if you're reading this and feel deflated or in a state of depression, especially if you've felt this way for a long time, my advice would be to at least have your blood tested, measuring your total and free testosterone levels. This should be the very minimum. If your results come back and you're in a healthy range, even high on the nmol scale, we can presume it's not your hormones causing your problems. We can at least advocate the process of elimination in your diagnosis, meaning we can focus on other aspects that may be causing your low mood, potentially; trauma, lifestyle, relationships, etc.

It's also possible that you may have low total testosterone but a high free-testosterone measurement. If this is the case and your primary goal is bodybuilding or working on your physique, I would advise against injecting external testosterone. Free testosterone is not bound to androgen receptors and is bio-available within our systems, enabling us to build muscle, burn fat, etc. So, if you're high in free testosterone but low in total testosterone, I wouldn't worry too much if you're more physique orientated. Too much testosterone converts to oestrogen through dihydrotestosterone (DHT) and the aromatase enzyme, but that's another topic, for another time. We just want to focus on healthy, therapeutic levels of testosterone.

Lastly, I just want to note depression and any feelings of deflation that may have led you to purchase this book, it's cliché, but things can improve. A few years back, I had moved out of my mother's home and worked hundreds of miles away in the UK. I didn't have many friends, and I spent a lot of my time reading, watching movies, etc. Something you have probably done yourself many times. However, this enabled me to recognise that you can put an indent in loneliness by surrounding yourself with positive people. By surrounding yourself with at least five positive personalities, can significantly help overcome feelings of loneliness. These personalities can come in the form of authors, characters on YouTube, anything, or anyone you can identify with or make a connection with. Also, many social forums and applications are designed to combat loneliness, as many are in the same situations.

I'd like to finally state that if you can find hope of some sort, or a purpose, this will be massively beneficial. Having hope and something to aim for, as cliché as it sounds, is not to be underestimated. We are only on this planet for a finite amount of time, and it's up to us to make the most of our existence. You could aim to learn a new skill, dedicate yourself to a new craft, and eventually, you will become proficient in that particular discipline; this is very possible. One book that has helped me is Man's Search for Meaning by Viktor Frankl. I won't give away too much, but if a man can find purpose in Frankl's circumstances, this enables hope for anyone suffering, and I remain optimistic that, you the reader, will find hope & purpose also.

RECOMMENDATIONS

Finally, a few recommendations from myself are people's personal anecdotal experiences you can follow. I implore you to investigate the following YouTube channels where patients on TRT (testosterone replacement therapy) have documented their experiences. Some of these are also below are also endocrine specialists such as Dr. Rand on Muscle Insider; these channels are:
- BigOKnow
- Paulo Broccardo
- Anabolic Doc
- Muscle Insider
- Jay Campbell

Once again, thank you for purchasing this book. If you would like to be notified of future books released, then please join our community by following the steps at the beginning of the book. We have a Facebook group with almost 1000 members who all help one another; we focus on techniques to improve cognitive abilities and new ways to learn new skills, everyone is welcome! I will be looking to go on TRT myself, so please subscribe to follow my journey and see my progress.

SOURCES

Ben. (2021, March 30). *Suicide is the single biggest killer of men under 45*. https://ben.org.uk/ourservices/healthandwellbeing/topsearches/menshealth/suicide/

Davis, N. (2018, November 14). *Testosterone therapy could help tackle depression in men – study*. The Guardian. https://www.theguardian.com/society/2018/nov/14/testosterone-therapy-could-help-tackle-male-depression-study

Engelson, E. S., Rabkin, J. G., Rabkin, R., & Kotler, D. P. (1996). Effects of Testosterone upon Body Composition. *Journal of Acquired Immune Deficiency Syndromes and Human Retrovirology*, *11*(5), 510. https://doi.org/10.1097/00042560-199604150-00012

Harvard Health Publishing. (2008). *Testosterone, aging, and the mind*. Harvard Health. https://www.health.harvard.edu/newsletter_article/Testosterone_aging_and_the_mind

Kocsis, M. (2021, March 14). *What are normal testosterone levels?* Balance My Hormones. https://balancemyhormones.co.uk/what-are-normal-testosterone-levels/#Normal_testosterone_levels_in_men_and_women_Adults

Lauren. (2020, October 30). *Six Ways To Increase Testosterone Naturally | Nature Cure Family Health - Tucson, AZ*. Nature

Cure Family Health. https://www.naturecurefamilyhealth.com/articles/six-ways-to-increase-testosterone-naturally/

Pizzorno L. (2015). Nothing Boring About Boron. *Integrative medicine (Encinitas, Calif.)*, *14*(4), 35–48.

Preti, A. (2003). Unemployment and suicide. *Journal of Epidemiology & Community Health*, *57*(8), 557–558. https://doi.org/10.1136/jech.57.8.557

Riumallo-Herl, C., Basu, S., Stuckler, D., Courtin, E., & Avendano, M. (2014). Job loss, wealth and depression during the Great Recession in the USA and Europe. *International Journal of Epidemiology*, *43*(5), 1508–1517. https://doi.org/10.1093/ije/dyu048

Suicide facts and figures. (2020). Samaritans. https://www.samaritans.org/about-samaritans/research-policy/suicide-facts-and-figures/.

TRADING ECONOMICS | 300.00 INDICATORS | 196 COUNTRIES. (2019). Trading Economics. https://tradingeconomics.com/united-kingdom/unemployment-rate

Yau, E. (2018, June 23). *Why suicide is more common among celebrities, CEOs and creatives, and how therapy helps*. South China Morning Post. https://www.scmp.com/lifestyle/health-wellness/article/2151761/why-suicide-more-common-among-celebrities-ceos-and

Walther, A., Breidenstein, J., & Miller, R. (2019). Association of Testosterone Treatment With Alleviation of

Depressive Symptoms in Men. *JAMA Psychiatry*, *76*(1), 31. https://doi.org/10.1001/jamapsychiatry.2018.2734